A
PILLOW STREWED
WITH THORNS

POETRY OF
SLEEPLESS NIGHTS
WRITTEN BY FAMED AUTHORS

By

VARIOUS

Read & Co.

Copyright © 2020 Ragged Hand

This edition is published by Ragged Hand,
an imprint of Read & Co.

This book is copyright and may not be reproduced or copied in any
way without the express permission of the publisher in writing.

British Library Cataloguing-in-Publication Data
A catalogue record for this book is available
from the British Library.

Read & Co. is part of Read Books Ltd.
For more information visit
www.readandcobooks.co.uk

"a pillow strewed with thorns"

—JANE AUSTEN
Northanger Abbey, 1817

CONTENTS

"During last night's insomnia, as these thoughts came and went between my aching temples, I realised once again, what I had almost forgotten in this recent period of relative calm, that I tread a terribly tenuous, indeed almost non-existent soil spread over a pit full of shadows, whence the powers of darkness emerge at will to destroy my life…"

—FRANZ KAFKA

"Every man's insomnia is as different from his neighbor's as are their daytime hopes and aspirations."

— F. Scott Fitzgerald

"But his dread was the nights when he could not sleep. Then it was awful indeed, when annihilation pressed in on him on every side. Then it was ghastly, to exist without having any life: lifeless, in the night, to exist."

— D. H. LAWRENCE

A
PILLOW STREWED
WITH THORNS

POETRY ON SLEEPLESSNESS

BELLS IN THE RAIN

By Elinor Wylie

Sleep falls, with limpid drops of rain,
Upon the steep cliffs of the town.
Sleep falls; men are at peace again
Awhile the small drops fall softly down.

The bright drops ring like bells of glass
Thinned by the wind, and lightly blown;
Sleep cannot fall on peaceful grass
So softly as it falls on stone.

Peace falls unheeded on the dead
Asleep; they have had deep peace to drink;
Upon a live man's bloody head
It falls most tenderly, I think.

FIRST PUBLISHED IN
Nets to Catch the Wind, 1921

SUNSET ON THE SPIRE

By Elinor Wylie

All that I dream
    By day or night
Lives in that stream
    Of lovely light.
Here is the earth,
    And there is the spire;
This is my hearth,
    And that is my fire.
From the sun's dome
    I am shouted proof
That this is my home,
    And that is my roof.
Here is my food,
    And here is my drink,
And I am wooed
    From the moon's brink.
And the days go over,
    And the nights end;
Here is my lover,
    Here is my friend
All that I
    Could ever ask
Wears that sky
    Like a thin gold mask.

FIRST PUBLISHED IN
Collected Poems of Elinor Wylie, 1932

INSOMNIA

By Dante Gabriel Rossetti

Thin are the night-skirts left behind
By daybreak hours that onward creep,
And thin, alas! the shred of sleep
That wavers with the spirit's wind:
But in half-dreams that shift and roll
And still remember and forget,
My soul this hour has drawn your soul
A little nearer yet.

Our lives, most dear, are never near,
Our thoughts are never far apart,
Though all that draws us heart to heart
Seems fainter now and now more clear.
To-night Love claims his full control,
And with desire and with regret
My soul this hour has drawn your soul
A little nearer yet.

Is there a home where heavy earth
Melts to bright air that breathes no pain,
Where water leaves no thirst again
And springing fire is Love's new birth?
If faith long bound to one true goal
May there at length its hope beget,
My soul that hour shall draw your soul
For ever nearer yet.

FIRST PUBLISHED IN
Ballads and Sonnets, 1881

THE SLEEPERS

By Walt Whitman

1

I wander all night in my vision,
Stepping with light feet, swiftly and noiselessly stepping and
stopping,
Bending with open eyes over the shut eyes of sleepers,
Wandering and confused, lost to myself, ill-assorted, contradictory,
Pausing, gazing, bending, and stopping.

How solemn they look there, stretch'd and still,
How quiet they breathe, the little children in their cradles.

The wretched features of ennuyes, the white features of corpses, the
livid faces of drunkards, the sick-gray faces of onanists,
The gash'd bodies on battle-fields, the insane in their strong-door'd
rooms, the sacred idiots, the new-born emerging
from gates, and the dying emerging from gates,
The night pervades them and infolds them.

The married couple sleep calmly in their bed, he with his palm
on the hip of the wife, and she with her palm on the hip of the
husband,
The sisters sleep lovingly side by side in their bed,
The men sleep lovingly side by side in theirs,
And the mother sleeps with her little child carefully wrapt.

The blind sleep, and the deaf and dumb sleep,
The prisoner sleeps well in the prison, the runaway son sleeps,
The murderer that is to be hung next day, how does he sleep?
And the murder'd person, how does he sleep?

The female that loves unrequited sleeps,
And the male that loves unrequited sleeps,
The head of the money-maker that plotted all day sleeps,
And the enraged and treacherous dispositions, all, all sleep.

I stand in the dark with drooping eyes by the worst-suffering
and the most restless,
I pass my hands soothingly to and fro a few inches from them,
The restless sink in their beds, they fitfully sleep.

Now I pierce the darkness, new beings appear,
The earth recedes from me into the night,
I saw that it was beautiful, and I see that what is not the earth is
beautiful.

I go from bedside to bedside, I sleep close with the other
sleepers each in turn,
I dream in my dream all the dreams of the other dreamers,
And I become the other dreamers.

I am a dance—play up there! the fit is whirling me fast!

I am the ever-laughing—it is new moon and twilight,
I see the hiding of douceurs, I see nimble ghosts whichever way
I look,
Cache and cache again deep in the ground and sea, and where
it is neither ground nor sea.

Well do they do their jobs those journeymen divine,

Only from me can they hide nothing, and would not if they could,
I reckon I am their boss and they make me a pet besides,
And surround me and lead me and run ahead when I walk,
To lift their cunning covers to signify me with stretch'd arms, and
resume the way;
Onward we move, a gay gang of blackguards! with mirth-shouting
music and wild-flapping pennants of joy!

I am the actor, the actress, the voter, the politician,
The emigrant and the exile, the criminal that stood in the box,
He who has been famous and he who shall be famous after to-day,
The stammerer, the well-form'd person, the wasted or feeble person.

I am she who adorn'd herself and folded her hair expectantly,
My truant lover has come, and it is dark.

Double yourself and receive me darkness,
Receive me and my lover too, he will not let me go without him.

I roll myself upon you as upon a bed, I resign myself to the dusk.

He whom I call answers me and takes the place of my lover,
He rises with me silently from the bed.

Darkness, you are gentler than my lover, his flesh was sweaty and
panting,
I feel the hot moisture yet that he left me.

My hands are spread forth, I pass them in all directions,
I would sound up the shadowy shore to which you are journeying.

Be careful darkness! already what was it touch'd me?
I thought my lover had gone, else darkness and he are one,
I hear the heart-beat, I follow, I fade away.

2

I descend my western course, my sinews are flaccid,
Perfume and youth course through me and I am their wake.

It is my face yellow and wrinkled instead of the old woman's,
I sit low in a straw-bottom chair and carefully darn my
grandson's stockings.

It is I too, the sleepless widow looking out on the winter
midnight,
I see the sparkles of starshine on the icy and pallid earth.

A shroud I see and I am the shroud, I wrap a body and lie in the
coffin,
It is dark here under ground, it is not evil or pain here, it is blank
here, for reasons.

(It seems to me that every thing in the light and air ought to be
happy,
Whoever is not in his coffin and the dark grave let him know he
has enough.)

3

I see a beautiful gigantic swimmer swimming naked through the
eddies of the sea,
His brown hair lies close and even to his head, he strikes out with
courageous arms, he urges himself with his legs,
I see his white body, I see his undaunted eyes,
I hate the swift-running eddies that would dash him head-
foremost on the rocks.

What are you doing you ruffianly red-trickled waves?

Will you kill the courageous giant? will you kill him in the prime of
his middle age?

Steady and long he struggles,
He is baffled, bang'd, bruis'd, he holds out while his strength holds
out,
The slapping eddies are spotted with his blood, they bear him away,
they roll him, swing him, turn him,
His beautiful body is borne in the circling eddies, it is continually
bruis'd on rocks,
Swiftly and ought of sight is borne the brave corpse.

4

I turn but do not extricate myself,
Confused, a past-reading, another, but with darkness yet.

The beach is cut by the razory ice-wind, the wreck-guns sound,
The tempest lulls, the moon comes floundering through the drifts.

I look where the ship helplessly heads end on, I hear the burst as she
strikes, I hear the howls of dismay, they grow fainter and fainter.

I cannot aid with my wringing fingers,
I can but rush to the surf and let it drench me and freeze upon me.

I search with the crowd, not one of the company is wash'd to us
alive,
In the morning I help pick up the dead and lay them in rows in a
barn.

5

Now of the older war-days, the defeat at Brooklyn,
Washington stands inside the lines, he stands on the intrench'd
hills amid a crowd of officers.
His face is cold and damp, he cannot repress the weeping drops,
He lifts the glass perpetually to his eyes, the color is blanch'd
from his cheeks,
He sees the slaughter of the southern braves confided to him by
their parents.

The same at last and at last when peace is declared,
He stands in the room of the old tavern, the well-belov'd soldiers
all pass through,
The officers speechless and slow draw near in their turns,
The chief encircles their necks with his arm and kisses them on
the cheek,
He kisses lightly the wet cheeks one after another, he shakes
hands and bids good-by to the army.

6

Now what my mother told me one day as we sat at dinner
together,
Of when she was a nearly grown girl living home with her
parents on the old homestead.

A red squaw came one breakfast-time to the old homestead,
On her back she carried a bundle of rushes for rush-bottoming
chairs,
Her hair, straight, shiny, coarse, black, profuse, half-envelop'd
her face,
Her step was free and elastic, and her voice sounded exquisitely
as she spoke.

My mother look'd in delight and amazement at the stranger,
She look'd at the freshness of her tall-borne face and full and
pliant limbs,
The more she look'd upon her she loved her,
Never before had she seen such wonderful beauty and purity,
She made her sit on a bench by the jamb of the fireplace, she
cook'd food for her,
She had no work to give her, but she gave her remembrance and
fondness.

The red squaw staid all the forenoon, and toward the middle of
the afternoon she went away,
O my mother was loth to have her go away,
All the week she thought of her, she watch'd for her many a
month,
She remember'd her many a winter and many a summer,
But the red squaw never came nor was heard of there again.

7

A show of the summer softness—a contact of something
unseen—an amour of the light and air,
I am jealous and overwhelm'd with friendliness,
And will go gallivant with the light and air myself.

O love and summer, you are in the dreams and in me,
Autumn and winter are in the dreams, the farmer goes with his
thrift,
The droves and crops increase, the barns are well-fill'd.

Elements merge in the night, ships make tacks in the dreams,
The sailor sails, the exile returns home,

The fugitive returns unharm'd, the immigrant is back beyond
months and years,
The poor Irishman lives in the simple house of his childhood with
the well known neighbors and faces,
They warmly welcome him, he is barefoot again, he forgets he is
well off,
The Dutchman voyages home, and the Scotchman and Welshman
voyage home, and the native of the Mediterranean voyages home,
To every port of England, France, Spain, enter well-fill'd ships,
The Swiss foots it toward his hills, the Prussian goes his way, the
Hungarian his way, and the Pole his way,
The Swede returns, and the Dane and Norwegian return.

The homeward bound and the outward bound,
The beautiful lost swimmer, the ennuye, the onanist, the female
that loves unrequited, the money-maker,
The actor and actress, those through with their parts and those
waiting to commence,
The affectionate boy, the husband and wife, the voter, the nominee
that is chosen and the nominee that has fail'd,
The great already known and the great any time after to-day,
The stammerer, the sick, the perfect-form'd, the homely,
The criminal that stood in the box, the judge that sat and
sentenced him, the fluent lawyers, the jury, the audience,
The laugher and weeper, the dancer, the midnight widow, the red
squaw,
The consumptive, the erysipalite, the idiot, he that is wrong'd,
The antipodes, and every one between this and them in the dark,
I swear they are averaged now—one is no better than the other,
The night and sleep have liken'd them and restored them.

I swear they are all beautiful,
Every one that sleeps is beautiful, every thing in the dim light is
beautiful,
The wildest and bloodiest is over, and all is peace.

Peace is always beautiful,
The myth of heaven indicates peace and night.

The myth of heaven indicates the soul,
The soul is always beautiful, it appears more or it appears less, it comes or it lags behind,
It comes from its embower'd garden and looks pleasantly on itself and encloses the world,
Perfect and clean the genitals previously jetting,and perfect and clean the womb cohering,
The head well-grown proportion'd and plumb, and the bowels and joints proportion'd and plumb.

The soul is always beautiful,
The universe is duly in order, every thing is in its place,
What has arrived is in its place and what waits shall be in its place,
The twisted skull waits, the watery or rotten blood waits,
The child of the glutton or venerealee waits long, and the child of the drunkard waits long, and the drunkard himself waits long,
The sleepers that lived and died wait, the far advanced are to go on in their turns, and the far behind are to come on in their turns,
The diverse shall be no less diverse, but they shall flow and unite— they unite now.

8

The sleepers are very beautiful as they lie unclothed,
They flow hand in hand over the whole earth from east to west as they lie unclothed,
The Asiatic and African are hand in hand, the European and American are hand in hand,
Learn'd and unlearn'd are hand in hand, and male and female are hand in hand,

The bare arm of the girl crosses the bare breast of her lover, they
press close without lust, his lips press her neck,
The father holds his grown or ungrown son in his arms with
measureless love, and the son holds the father in his arms with
measureless love,
The white hair of the mother shines on the white wrist of the
daughter,
The breath of the boy goes with the breath of the man, friend is
inarm'd by friend,
The scholar kisses the teacher and the teacher kisses the scholar,
the wrong 'd made right,
The call of the slave is one with the master's call, and the master
salutes the slave,
The felon steps forth from the prison, the insane becomes sane, the
suffering of sick persons is reliev'd,
The sweatings and fevers stop, the throat that was unsound
is sound, the lungs of the consumptive are resumed, the poor
distress'd head is free,
The joints of the rheumatic move as smoothly as ever, and
smoother than ever,
Stiflings and passages open, the paralyzed become supple,
The swell'd and convuls'd and congested awake to themselves in
condition,
They pass the invigoration of the night and the chemistry of the
night, and awake.

I too pass from the night,
I stay a while away O night, but I return to you again and love you.

Why should I be afraid to trust myself to you?
I am not afraid, I have been well brought forward by you,
I love the rich running day, but I do not desert her in whom I lay
so long,

I know not how I came of you and I know not where I go with
you, but
I know I came well and shall go well.

I will stop only a time with the night, and rise betimes,
I will duly pass the day O my mother, and duly return to you.

ORIGINALLY CALLED
Night Poem in 1856 and then *Sleep-Chasings* in 1860.

HOURS CONTINUING LONG

By Walt Whitman

HOURS continuing long, sore and heavy-hearted,
Hours of the dusk, when I withdraw to a lonesome and
unfrequented spot, seating myself, leaning my face in my
hands;
Hours sleepless, deep in the night, when I go forth, speeding
swiftly the country roads, or through the city streets, or pacing
miles and miles, stifling plaintive cries;
Hours discouraged, distracted—for the one I cannot content
myself without, soon I saw him content himself without me;
Hours when I am forgotten, (O weeks and months are passing,
but I believe I am never to forget!)
Sullen and suffering hours! (I am ashamed—but it is useless—I
am what I am;)
Hours of my torment—I wonder if other men ever have the like,
out of the like feelings?
Is there even one other like me—distracted—his friend, his
lover, lost to him?
Is he too as I am now? Does he still rise in the morning,
dejected, thinking who is lost to him? and at night, awaking,
think who is lost?
Does he too harbor his friendship silent and endless? harbor his
anguish and passion?
Does some stray reminder, or the casual mention of a name,
bring the fit back upon him, taciturn and deprest?

Does he see himself reflected in me? In these hours,
does he see the face of his hours reflected?

FIRST PUBLISHED IN
Leaves, 1860 as *Calamus*

TO SLEEP

By William Wordsworth

A flock of sheep that leisurely pass by
    One after one; the sound of rain, and bees
    Murmuring; the fall of rivers, winds and seas,
Smooth fields, white sheets of water, and pure sky —

I've thought of all by turns, and still I lie
    Sleepless; and soon the small birds' melodies
    Must hear, first utter'd from my orchard trees,
And the first cuckoo's melancholy cry.

Even thus last night, and two nights more I lay,
    And could not win thee, Sleep, by any stealth:
So do not let me wear to-night away.
    Without thee what is all the morning's wealth?
Come, blessed barrier between day and day,
Dear mother of fresh thoughts and joyous health!

FIRST PUBLISHED IN
Poems - Volume II, 1815

ASTROPHIL AND STELLA 39

COME SLEEP!
O SLEEP, THE CERTAIN KNOT OF PEACE

By Sir Philip Sidney

Come Sleep! O Sleep, the certain knot of peace,
The baiting-place of wit, the balm of woe,
The poor man's wealth, the prisoner's release,
Th' indifferent judge between the high and low.
With shield of proof shield me from out the prease
Of those fierce darts despair at me doth throw:
O make in me those civil wars to cease;
I will good tribute pay, if thou do so.
Take thou of me smooth pillows, sweetest bed,
A chamber deaf to noise and blind to light,
A rosy garland and a weary head:
And if these things, as being thine by right,
Move not thy heavy grace, thou shalt in me,
Livelier than elsewhere, Stella's image see.

FIRST PUBLISHED IN
Astrophil and Stella, 1591

SONNET 27

_____

By William Shakespeare

Weary with toil, I haste me to my bed,
The dear repose for limbs with travel tired;
But then begins a journey in my head,
To work my mind, when body's work's expired:
For then my thoughts (from far where I abide)
Intend a zealous pilgrimage to thee,
And keep my drooping eyelids open wide,
Looking on darkness which the blind do see:
Save that my soul's imaginary sight
Presents thy shadow to my sightless view,
Which, like a jewel hung in ghastly night,
Makes black night beauteous and her old face new.
  Lo, thus, by day my limbs, by night my mind,
  For thee, and for myself, no quiet find.

FIRST PUBLISHED IN
Shakespeare's Sonnets, 1609

THE FIRST PART

SONNET 9

By William Drummond

SLEEP, Silence' child, sweet father of soft rest,
Prince, whose approach peace to all mortals brings,
Indifferent host to shepherds and to kings,
Sole comforter of minds with grief oppressed;
Lo, by thy charming rod all breathing things
Lie slumb'ring, with forgetfulness possessed,
And yet o'er me to spread thy drowsy wings
Thou spar'st, alas! who cannot be thy guest.
Since I am thine, O come, but with that face
To inward light which thou art wont to show,
With feigned solace ease a true-felt woe;
Or if, deaf god, thou do deny that grace,
   Come as thou wilt, and what thou wilt bequeath,
   I long to kiss the image of my death.

A SONNET FROM
*The Poetical Works of William
Drummond of Hawthornden*, 1913

THE LOVER TO HIS BED, WITH DESCRIBING OF HIS UNQUIET STATE

By Sir Thomas Wyatt

THE RESTFUL place, renewer of my smart,
The labours' salve, increasing my sorrow,
The body's ease, and troubler of my heart,
Quieter of mind, mine unquiet foe,
Forgetter of pain, rememberer of my woe,
The place of sleep, wherein I do but wake,
Besprent with tears, my bed, I thee forsake.
   The frosty snows may not redress my heat,
Nor heat of sun abate my fervent cold,
I know nothing to ease my pains so great;
Each cure causeth increase by twenty fold,
Renewing cares upon my sorrows old,
Such overthwart effects in me they make:
Besprent with tears, my bed for to forsake.
   But all for nought, I find no better ease
In bed or out: this most causeth my pain,
Where I do seek how best that I may please;
My lost labour, alas, is all in vain:
My heart once set, I cannot it refrain;
No place from me my grief away can take;
Wherefore with tears, my bed, I thee forsake.

FIRST PUBLISHED IN
The poetical works of Sir Thomas Wyatt, Odes, 1854

OF CONSCIOUSNESS,
HER AWFUL MATE

By Emily Dickinson

Of Consciousness, her awful Mate
The Soul cannot be rid —
As easy the secreting her
Behind the Eyes of God.

The deepest hid is sighted first
And scant to Him the Crowd —
What triple Lenses burn upon
The Escapade from God —

A POEM FROM
Poems by Emily Dickinson, 1890

IT WAS GIVEN TO ME BY THE GODS

By Emily Dickinson

It was given to me by the Gods—
When I was a little Girl—
They given us Presents most—you know—
When we are new—and small.
I kept it in my Hand—
I never put it down—
I did not dare to eat—or sleep—
For fear it would be gone—
I heard such words as "Rich"—
When hurrying to school—
From lips at Corners of the Streets—
And wrestled with a smile.
Rich! 'Twas Myself—was rich—
To take the name of Gold—
And Gold to own—in solid Bars—
The Difference—made me bold—

ORIGINALLY IN
Packet XXXIV, Fascicle 21, 1862
FIRST PUBLISHED IN
Bolts of Melody, 1945

WATER
MAKES MANY BEDS

By Emily Dickinson

Water makes many Beds
For those averse to sleep—
Its awful chamber open stands—
Its Curtains blandly sweep—
Abhorrent is the Rest
In undulating Rooms
Whose Amplitude no end invades—
Whose Axis never comes.

FIRST PUBLISHED IN 1877

A SPIDER
SEWED AT NIGHT

By Emily Dickinson

A Spider sewed at Night
Without a Light
Upon an Arc of White.

If Ruff it was of Dame
Or Shroud of Gnome
Himself himself inform.

Of Immortality
His Strategy
Was Physiognomy.

A POEM FROM
Complete Poems, Part Two, 1924

SLEEP IS
SUPPOSED TO BE

By Emily Dickinson

Sleep is supposed to be,
By souls of sanity,
The shutting of the eye.

Sleep is the station grand
Down which on either hand
The hosts of witness stand!

A POEM FROM
Complete Poems, Part Four, 1924

SLEEP BRINGS NO JOY TO ME

By Emily Brontë

XIV

Sleep brings no joy to me,
  Remembrance never dies,
My soul is given to mystery,
  And lives in sighs.

Sleep brings no rest to me;
  The shadows of the dead,
My wakening eyes may never see,
  Surround my bed.

Sleep brings no hope to me,
  In soundest sleep they come,
And with their doleful imag'ry
  Deepen the gloom.

Sleep brings no strength to me,
  No power renewed to brave;
I only sail a wilder sea,
  A darker wave.

Sleep brings no friend to me
  To soothe and aid to bear;
They all gaze on how scornfully,
  And I despair.

Sleep brings no wish to fret
  My harassed heart beneath;
My only wish is to forget
  In endless sleep of death.

November 1837

A POEM FROM
Poems by Charlotte,
Emily, and Anne Brontë, 1902

STARS

By Emily Brontë

Ah! why, because the dazzling sun
Restored my earth to joy
Have you departed, every one,
And left a desert sky?

All through the night, your glorious eyes
Were gazing down in mine,
And with a full heart's thankful sighs
I blessed that watch divine!

I was at peace, and drank your beams
As they were life to me
And revelled in my changeful dreams
Like petrel on the sea.

Thought followed thought—star followed star
Through boundless regions on,
While one sweet influence, near and far,
Thrilled through and proved us one.

Why did the morning rise to break
So great, so pure a spell,
And scorch with fire the tranquil cheek
Where your cool radiance fell?

Blood-red he rose, and arrow-straight,
His fierce beams struck my brow;
The soul of Nature sprang elate,
But mine sank sad and low!

My lids closed down—yet through their veil
I saw him blazing still;
And bathe in gold the misty dale,
And flash upon the hill.

I turned me to the pillow then
To call back Night, and see
Your worlds of solemn light, again
Throb with my heart and me!

It would not do—the pillow glowed
And glowed both roof and floor,
And birds sang loudly in the wood,
And fresh winds shook the door.

The curtains waved, the wakened flies
Were murmuring round my room,
Imprisoned there, till I should rise
And give them leave to roam.

O Stars and Dreams and Gentle Night;
O Night and Stars return!
And hide me from the hostile light
That does not warm, but burn—

That drains the blood of suffering men;
Drinks tears, instead of dew:
Let me sleep through his blinding reign,
And only wake with you!

FIRST PUBLISHED IN
Poems by Currer, Ellis, and Acton Bell, 1846

IN MEMORIAM

AN EXCERPT

By Alfred Lord Tennyson

VII

Dark house, by which once more I stand
  Here in the long unlovely street,
  Doors, where my heart was used to beat
So quickly, waiting for a hand,

A hand that can be clasp'd no more—
  Behold me, for I cannot sleep,
  And like a guilty thing I creep
At earliest morning to the door.

He is not here; but far away
  The noise of life begins again,
  And ghastly thro' the drizzling rain
On the bald street breaks the blank day.

FIRST PUBLISHED IN
In Memoriam, 1850

INSOMNIA

By John B. Tabb

E'en this, Lord, didst thou bless —
This pain of sleeplessness —
　　The livelong night,
Urging God's gentlest angel from thy side,
That anguish only might with thee abide
　　Until the light.
Yea, e'en the last and best,
Thy victory and rest,
　　Came thus to thee;
For't was while others calmly slept around,
That thou alone in sleeplessness wast found,
　　To comfort me.

FIRST PUBLISHED IN
Lyrics, 1897

SLEEP

By John B. Tabb

What art thou, balmy sleep?
"Foam from the fragrant deep
Of silence, hither blown
From the hushed waves of tone."

FIRST PUBLISHED IN
Poems, 1894

SLUMBER - SONG

By John B. Tabb

Sleep! The spirits that attend
On thy waking hours are fled.
Heaven thou canst not now offend
Till thy slumber-plumes are shed;
Consciousness alone doth lend
Life its pain, and Death its dread;
Innocence and Peace befriend
All the sleeping and the dead.

FIRST PUBLISHED IN
Lyrics, 1897

DAWN

By John B. Tabb

Behold, as from a silver-horn,
The sacerdotal Night
Outpours upon his latest-born
The chrism of the light;
And bids him to the alter come,
Whereon for sacrifice,
(A lamb before his shearers, dumb,)
A victim shadow lies.

FIRST PUBLISHED IN
Lyrics, 1897

THE TRIUMPH OF LIFE

By Percy Bysshe Shelley

Swift as a spirit hastening to his task
Of glory and of good, the Sun sprang forth
Rejoicing in his splendour, and the mask

Of darkness fell from the awakened Earth—
The smokeless altars of the mountain snows
Flamed above crimson clouds, and at the birth

Of light, the Ocean's orison arose,
To which the birds tempered their matin lay.
All flowers in field or forest which unclose

Their trembling eyelids to the kiss of day,
Swinging their censers in the element,
With orient incense lit by the new ray

Burned slow and inconsumably, and sent
Their odorous sighs up to the smiling air;
And, in succession due, did continent,

Isle, ocean, and all things that in them wear
The form and character of mortal mould,
Rise as the Sun their father rose, to bear

Their portion of the toil, which he of old
Took as his own, and then imposed on them:
But I, whom thoughts which must remain untold

Had kept as wakeful as the stars that gem
The cone of night, now they were laid asleep
Stretched my faint limbs beneath the hoary stem

Which an old chestnut flung athwart the steep
Of a green Apennine: before me fled
The night; behind me rose the day; the deep

Was at my feet, and Heaven above my head,—
When a strange trance over my fancy grew
Which was not slumber, for the shade it spread

Was so transparent, that the scene came through
As clear as when a veil of light is drawn
O'er evening hills they glimmer; and I knew

That I had felt the freshness of that dawn
Bathe in the same cold dew my brow and hair,
And sate as thus upon that slope of lawn

Under the self-same bough, and heard as there
The birds, the fountains and the ocean hold
Sweet talk in music through the enamoured air,
And then a vision on my train was rolled.

. . .

As in that trance of wondrous thought I lay,
This was the tenour of my waking dream:—
Methought I sate beside a public way

Thick strewn with summer dust, and a great stream
Of people there was hurrying to and fro,
Numerous as gnats upon the evening gleam,

All hastening onward, yet none seemed to know
Whither he went, or whence he came, or why
He made one of the multitude, and so

Was borne amid the crowd, as through the sky
One of the million leaves of summer's bier;
Old age and youth, manhood and infancy,

Mixed in one mighty torrent did appear,
Some flying from the thing they feared, and some
Seeking the object of another's fear;

And others, as with steps towards the tomb,
Pored on the trodden worms that crawled beneath,
And others mournfully within the gloom

Of their own shadow walked, and called it death;
And some fled from it as it were a ghost,
Half fainting in the affliction of vain breath:

But more, with motions which each other crossed,
Pursued or shunned the shadows the clouds threw,
Or birds within the noonday aether lost,

Upon that path where flowers never grew,—
And, weary with vain toil and faint for thirst,
Heard not the fountains, whose melodious dew

Out of their mossy cells forever burst;
Nor felt the breeze which from the forest told
Of grassy paths and wood-lawns interspersed

54

With overarching elms and caverns cold,
And violet banks where sweet dreams brood, but they
Pursued their serious folly as of old.

And as I gazed, methought that in the way
The throng grew wilder, as the woods of June
When the south wind shakes the extinguished day,

And a cold glare, intenser than the noon,
But icy cold, obscured with blinding light
The sun, as he the stars. Like the young moon—

When on the sunlit limits of the night
Her white shell trembles amid crimson air,
And whilst the sleeping tempest gathers might—

Doth, as the herald of its coming, bear
The ghost of its dead mother, whose dim form
Bends in dark aether from her infant's chair,—

So came a chariot on the silent storm
Of its own rushing splendour, and a Shape
So sate within, as one whom years deform,

Beneath a dusky hood and double cape,
Crouching within the shadow of a tomb;
And o'er what seemed the head a cloud-like crape

Was bent, a dun and faint aethereal gloom
Tempering the light. Upon the chariot-beam
A Janus-visaged Shadow did assume

The guidance of that wonder-winged team;
The shapes which drew it in thick lightenings
Were lost:—I heard alone on the air's soft stream

The music of their ever-moving wings.
All the four faces of that Charioteer
Had their eyes banded; little profit brings

Speed in the van and blindness in the rear,
Nor then avail the beams that quench the sun,—
Or that with banded eyes could pierce the sphere

Of all that is, has been or will be done;
So ill was the car guided—but it passed
With solemn speed majestically on.

The crowd gave way, and I arose aghast,
Or seemed to rise, so mighty was the trance,
And saw, like clouds upon the thunder-blast,

The million with fierce song and maniac dance
Raging around—such seemed the jubilee
As when to greet some conqueror's advance

Imperial Rome poured forth her living sea
From senate-house, and forum, and theatre,
When . . . upon the free

Had bound a yoke, which soon they stooped to bear.
Nor wanted here the just similitude
Of a triumphal pageant, for where'er

The chariot rolled, a captive multitude
Was driven;—all those who had grown old in power
Or misery,—all who had their age subdued

By action or by suffering, and whose hour
Was drained to its last sand in weal or woe,
So that the trunk survived both fruit and flower;—

All those whose fame or infamy must grow
Till the great winter lay the form and name
Of this green earth with them for ever low;—

All but the sacred few who could not tame
Their spirits to the conquerors —but as soon
As they had touched the world with living flame,

Fled back like eagles to their native noon,
Or those who put aside the diadem
Of earthly thrones or gems...

Were there, of Athens or Jerusalem.
Were neither mid the mighty captives seen,
Nor mid the ribald crowd that followed them,

Nor those who went before fierce and obscene.
The wild dance maddens in the van, and those
Who lead it—fleet as shadows on the green,

Outspeed the chariot, and without repose
Mix with each other in tempestuous measure
To savage music, wilder as it grows,

They, tortured by their agonizing pleasure,
Convulsed and on the rapid whirlwinds spun
Of that fierce Spirit, whose unholy leisure

Was soothed by mischief since the world begun,
Throw back their heads and loose their streaming hair;
And in their dance round her who dims the sun,

Maidens and youths fling their wild arms in air
As their feet twinkle; they recede, and now
Bending within each other's atmosphere,

Kindle invisibly—and as they glow,
Like moths by light attracted and repelled,
Oft to their bright destruction come and go,

Till like two clouds into one vale impelled,
That shake the mountains when their lightnings mingle
And die in rain—the fiery band which held

Their natures, snaps—while the shock still may tingle
One falls and then another in the path
Senseless—nor is the desolation single,

Yet ere I can say WHERE—the chariot hath
Passed over them—nor other trace I find
But as of foam after the ocean's wrath

Is spent upon the desert shore;—behind,
Old men and women foully disarrayed,
Shake their gray hairs in the insulting wind,

And follow in the dance, with limbs decayed,
Seeking to reach the light which leaves them still
Farther behind and deeper in the shade.

But not the less with impotence of will
They wheel, though ghastly shadows interpose
Round them and round each other, and fulfil

Their work, and in the dust from whence they rose
Sink, and corruption veils them as they lie,
And past in these performs what ... in those.

Struck to the heart by this sad pageantry,
Half to myself I said—'And what is this?
Whose shape is that within the car? And why—'

I would have added—'is all here amiss?—'
But a voice answered—'Life!'—I turned, and knew
(O Heaven, have mercy on such wretchedness!)

That what I thought was an old root which grew
To strange distortion out of the hill side,
Was indeed one of those deluded crew,

And that the grass, which methought hung so wide
And white, was but his thin discoloured hair,
And that the holes he vainly sought to hide,

Were or had been eyes:—'If thou canst forbear
To join the dance, which I had well forborne,'
Said the grim Feature, of my thought aware,

'I will unfold that which to this deep scorn
Led me and my companions, and relate
The progress of the pageant since the morn;

'If thirst of knowledge shall not then abate,
Follow it thou even to the night, but I
Am weary.'—Then like one who with the weight

Of his own words is staggered, wearily
He paused; and ere he could resume, I cried:
'First, who art thou?'—'Before thy memory,

'I feared, loved, hated, suffered, did and died,
And if the spark with which Heaven lit my spirit
Had been with purer nutriment supplied,

'Corruption would not now thus much inherit
Of what was once Rousseau,—nor this disguise
Stain that which ought to have disdained to wear it;

'If I have been extinguished, yet there rise
A thousand beacons from the spark I bore'—
'And who are those chained to the car?'—'The wise,

'The great, the unforgotten,—they who wore
Mitres and helms and crowns, or wreaths of light,
Signs of thought's empire over thought—their lore

'Taught them not this, to know themselves; their might
Could not repress the mystery within,
And for the morn of truth they feigned, deep night

'Caught them ere evening.'—'Who is he with chin
Upon his breast, and hands crossed on his chain?'—
'The child of a fierce hour; he sought to win

'The world, and lost all that it did contain
Of greatness, in its hope destroyed; and more
Of fame and peace than virtue's self can gain

'Without the opportunity which bore
Him on its eagle pinions to the peak
From which a thousand climbers have before

'Fallen, as Napoleon fell.'—I felt my cheek
Alter, to see the shadow pass away,
Whose grasp had left the giant world so weak

That every pigmy kicked it as it lay;
And much I grieved to think how power and will
In opposition rule our mortal day,

And why God made irreconcilable
Good and the means of good; and for despair
I half disdained mine eyes' desire to fill

With the spent vision of the times that were
And scarce have ceased to be.—'Dost thou behold,'
Said my guide, 'those spoilers spoiled, Voltaire,

'Frederick, and Paul, Catherine, and Leopold,
And hoary anarchs, demagogues, and sage—
names which the world thinks always old,

'For in the battle Life and they did wage,
She remained conqueror. I was overcome
By my own heart alone, which neither age,

'Nor tears, nor infamy, nor now the tomb
Could temper to its object.'—'Let them pass,'
I cried, 'the world and its mysterious doom

'Is not so much more glorious than it was,
That I desire to worship those who drew
New figures on its false and fragile glass

'As the old faded.'—'Figures ever new
Rise on the bubble, paint them as you may;
We have but thrown, as those before us threw,

'Our shadows on it as it passed away.
But mark how chained to the triumphal chair
The mighty phantoms of an elder day;

'All that is mortal of great Plato there
Expiates the joy and woe his master knew not;
The star that ruled his doom was far too fair.

'And life, where long that flower of Heaven grew not,
Conquered that heart by love, which gold, or pain,
Or age, or sloth, or slavery could subdue not.

'And near him walk the ... twain,
The tutor and his pupil, whom Dominion
Followed as tame as vulture in a chain.

'The world was darkened beneath either pinion
Of him whom from the flock of conquerors
Fame singled out for her thunder-bearing minion;

'The other long outlived both woes and wars,
Throned in the thoughts of men, and still had kept
The jealous key of Truth's eternal doors,

'If Bacon's eagle spirit had not lept
Like lightning out of darkness—he compelled
The Proteus shape of Nature, as it slept

'To wake, and lead him to the caves that held
The treasure of the secrets of its reign.
See the great bards of elder time, who quelled

'The passions which they sung, as by their strain
May well be known: their living melody
Tempers its own contagion to the vein

'Of those who are infected with it—I
Have suffered what I wrote, or viler pain!
And so my words have seeds of misery—

'Even as the deeds of others, not as theirs.'
And then he pointed to a company,

'Midst whom I quickly recognized the heirs
Of Caesar's crime, from him to Constantine;
The anarch chiefs, whose force and murderous snares

Had founded many a sceptre-bearing line,
And spread the plague of gold and blood abroad:
And Gregory and John, and men divine,

Who rose like shadows between man and God;
Till that eclipse, still hanging over heaven,
Was worshipped by the world o'er which they strode,

For the true sun it quenched—'Their power was given
But to destroy,' replied the leader:—'I
Am one of those who have created, even

'If it be but a world of agony.'—
'Whence camest thou? and whither goest thou?
How did thy course begin?' I said, 'and why?

'Mine eyes are sick of this perpetual flow
Of people, and my heart sick of one sad thought—
Speak!'—'Whence I am, I partly seem to know,

'And how and by what paths I have been brought
To this dread pass, methinks even thou mayst guess;—
Why this should be, my mind can compass not;

'Whither the conqueror hurries me, still less;—
But follow thou, and from spectator turn
Actor or victim in this wretchedness,

'And what thou wouldst be taught I then may learn
From thee. Now listen:—In the April prime,
When all the forest-tips began to burn

'With kindling green, touched by the azure clime
Of the young season, I was laid asleep
Under a mountain, which from unknown time

'Had yawned into a cavern, high and deep;
And from it came a gentle rivulet,
Whose water, like clear air, in its calm sweep

'Bent the soft grass, and kept for ever wet
The stems of the sweet flowers, and filled the grove
With sounds, which whoso hears must needs forget

'All pleasure and all pain, all hate and love,
Which they had known before that hour of rest;
A sleeping mother then would dream not of

'Her only child who died upon the breast
At eventide—a king would mourn no more
The crown of which his brows were dispossessed

'When the sun lingered o'er his ocean floor
To gild his rival's new prosperity.
'Thou wouldst forget thus vainly to deplore

'Ills, which if ills can find no cure from thee,
The thought of which no other sleep will quell,
Nor other music blot from memory,

'So sweet and deep is the oblivious spell;
And whether life had been before that sleep
The Heaven which I imagine, or a Hell

'Like this harsh world in which I woke to weep,
I know not. I arose, and for a space
The scene of woods and waters seemed to keep,

Though it was now broad day, a gentle trace
Of light diviner than the common sun
Sheds on the common earth, and all the place

'Was filled with magic sounds woven into one
Oblivious melody, confusing sense
Amid the gliding waves and shadows dun;

'And, as I looked, the bright omnipresence
Of morning through the orient cavern flowed,
And the sun's image radiantly intense

'Burned on the waters of the well that glowed
Like gold, and threaded all the forest's maze
With winding paths of emerald fire; there stood

'Amid the sun, as he amid the blaze
Of his own glory, on the vibrating
Floor of the fountain, paved with flashing rays,

'A Shape all light, which with one hand did fling
Dew on the earth, as if she were the dawn,
And the invisible rain did ever sing

'A silver music on the mossy lawn;
And still before me on the dusky grass,
Iris her many-coloured scarf had drawn:

'In her right hand she bore a crystal glass,
Mantling with bright Nepenthe; the fierce splendour
Fell from her as she moved under the mass

'Of the deep cavern, and with palms so tender,
Their tread broke not the mirror of its billow,
Glided along the river, and did bend her

'Head under the dark boughs, till like a willow
Her fair hair swept the bosom of the stream
That whispered with delight to be its pillow.

'As one enamoured is upborne in dream
O'er lily-paven lakes, mid silver mist
To wondrous music, so this shape might seem

'Partly to tread the waves with feet which kissed
The dancing foam; partly to glide along
The air which roughened the moist amethyst,

'Or the faint morning beams that fell among
The trees, or the soft shadows of the trees;
And her feet, ever to the ceaseless song

'Of leaves, and winds, and waves, and birds, and bees,
And falling drops, moved in a measure new
Yet sweet, as on the summer evening breeze,

'Up from the lake a shape of golden dew
Between two rocks, athwart the rising moon,
Dances i' the wind, where never eagle flew;

'And still her feet, no less than the sweet tune
To which they moved, seemed as they moved to blot
The thoughts of him who gazed on them; and soon

'All that was, seemed as if it had been not;
And all the gazer's mind was strewn beneath
Her feet like embers; and she, thought by thought,

'Trampled its sparks into the dust of death
As day upon the threshold of the east
Treads out the lamps of night, until the breath

'Of darkness re-illumine even the least
Of heaven's living eyes—like day she came,
Making the night a dream; and ere she ceased

'To move, as one between desire and shame
Suspended, I said—If, as it doth seem,
Thou comest from the realm without a name

'Into this valley of perpetual dream,
Show whence I came, and where I am, and why—
Pass not away upon the passing stream.

'Arise and quench thy thirst, was her reply.
And as a shut lily stricken by the wand
Of dewy morning's vital alchemy,

'I rose; and, bending at her sweet command,
Touched with faint lips the cup she raised,
And suddenly my brain became as sand

'Where the first wave had more than half erased
The track of deer on desert Labrador;
Whilst the wolf, from which they fled amazed,

'Leaves his stamp visibly upon the shore,
Until the second bursts;—so on my sight
Burst a new vision, never seen before,

'And the fair shape waned in the coming light,
As veil by veil the silent splendour drops
From Lucifer, amid the chrysolite

'Of sunrise, ere it tinge the mountain-tops;
And as the presence of that fairest planet,
Although unseen, is felt by one who hopes

'That his day's path may end as he began it,
In that star's smile, whose light is like the scent
Of a jonquil when evening breezes fan it,

'Or the soft note in which his dear lament
The Brescian shepherd breathes, or the caress
That turned his weary slumber to content;

'So knew I in that light's severe excess
The presence of that Shape which on the stream
Moved, as I moved along the wilderness,

68

'More dimly than a day-appearing dream,
The host of a forgotten form of sleep;
A light of heaven, whose half-extinguished beam

'Through the sick day in which we wake to weep
Glimmers, for ever sought, for ever lost;
So did that shape its obscure tenour keep

'Beside my path, as silent as a ghost;
But the new Vision, and the cold bright car,
With solemn speed and stunning music, crossed

'The forest, and as if from some dread war
Triumphantly returning, the loud million
Fiercely extolled the fortune of her star.

'A moving arch of victory, the vermilion
And green and azure plumes of Iris had
Built high over her wind-winged pavilion,

'And underneath aethereal glory clad
The wilderness, and far before her flew
The tempest of the splendour, which forbade

'Shadow to fall from leaf and stone; the crew
Seemed in that light, like atomies to dance
Within a sunbeam;—some upon the new

'Embroidery of flowers, that did enhance
The grassy vesture of the desert, played,
Forgetful of the chariot's swift advance;

'Others stood gazing, till within the shade
Of the great mountain its light left them dim;
Others outspeeded it; and others made

'Circles around it, like the clouds that swim
Round the high moon in a bright sea of air;
And more did follow, with exulting hymn,

'The chariot and the captives fettered there:—
But all like bubbles on an eddying flood
Fell into the same track at last, and were

'Borne onward.—I among the multitude
Was swept—me, sweetest flowers delayed not long;
Me, not the shadow nor the solitude;

'Me, not that falling stream's Lethean song;
Me, not the phantom of that early Form
Which moved upon its motion—but among

'The thickest billows of that living storm
I plunged, and bared my bosom to the clime
Of that cold light, whose airs too soon deform.

'Before the chariot had begun to climb
The opposing steep of that mysterious dell,
Behold a wonder worthy of the rhyme

'Of him who from the lowest depths of hell,
Through every paradise and through all glory,
Love led serene, and who returned to tell

'The words of hate and awe; the wondrous story
How all things are transfigured except Love;
For deaf as is a sea, which wrath makes hoary,

'The world can hear not the sweet notes that move
The sphere whose light is melody to lovers—
A wonder worthy of his rhyme.—The grove

'Grew dense with shadows to its inmost covers,
The earth was gray with phantoms, and the air
Was peopled with dim forms, as when there hovers

'A flock of vampire-bats before the glare
Of the tropic sun, bringing, ere evening,
Strange night upon some Indian isle; —thus were

'Phantoms diffused around; and some did fling
Shadows of shadows, yet unlike themselves,
Behind them; some like eaglets on the wing

'Were lost in the white day; others like elves
Danced in a thousand unimagined shapes
Upon the sunny streams and grassy shelves;

'And others sate chattering like restless apes
On vulgar hands,...
Some made a cradle of the ermined capes

'Of kingly mantles; some across the tiar
Of pontiffs sate like vultures; others played
Under the crown which girt with empire

'A baby's or an idiot's brow, and made
Their nests in it. The old anatomies
Sate hatching their bare broods under the shade

'Of daemon wings, and laughed from their dead eyes
To reassume the delegated power,
Arrayed in which those worms did monarchize,

'Who made this earth their charnel. Others more
Humble, like falcons, sate upon the fist
Of common men, and round their heads did soar;

Or like small gnats and flies, as thick as mist
On evening marshes, thronged about the brow
Of lawyers, statesmen, priest and theorist;—

'And others, like discoloured flakes of snow
On fairest bosoms and the sunniest hair,
Fell, and were melted by the youthful glow

'Which they extinguished; and, like tears, they were
A veil to those from whose faint lids they rained
In drops of sorrow. I became aware

'Of whence those forms proceeded which thus stained
The track in which we moved. After brief space,
From every form the beauty slowly waned;

'From every firmest limb and fairest face
The strength and freshness fell like dust, and left
The action and the shape without the grace

'Of life. The marble brow of youth was cleft
With care; and in those eyes where once hope shone,
Desire, like a lioness bereft

'Of her last cub, glared ere it died; each one
Of that great crowd sent forth incessantly
These shadows, numerous as the dead leaves blown

'In autumn evening from a poplar tree.
Each like himself and like each other were
At first; but some distorted seemed to be

'Obscure clouds, moulded by the casual air;
And of this stuff the car's creative ray
Wrought all the busy phantoms that were there,

'As the sun shapes the clouds; thus on the way
Mask after mask fell from the countenance
And form of all; and long before the day

'Was old, the joy which waked like heaven's glance
The sleepers in the oblivious valley, died;
And some grew weary of the ghastly dance,

'And fell, as I have fallen, by the wayside;—
Those soonest from whose forms most shadows passed,
And least of strength and beauty did abide.

'Then, what is life? I cried.'—

FIRST PUBLISHED IN
Posthumous Poems, 1824.

73

HUMANITAD

———————————————

AN EXCERPT

By Oscar Wilde

Nay! for perchance that poppy-crowned god
Is like the watcher by a sick man's bed
Who talks of sleep but gives it not; his rod
Hath lost its virtue, and, when all is said,
Death is too rude, too obvious a key
To solve one single secret in a life's philosophy.

FIRST PUBLISHED IN
Humanitad, 1890